Dedicated to Pastor Tim Jackson

Thank you for learning to love
yourself enough to get healthy.
You will be missed!

Coach

FOR

Nikolas and Kristopher.

I want you to understand how imperative it is to love yourself and know what that means. I share this book with you to bring awareness to your choices, feelings, and self. The choices you make now will set the course for the rest of your life. I want you both to learn to love the skin you're in, forgive yourself when you make a mistake, and have a genuine compassion toward others.

The love I have in my heart for both of you goes beyond the ends of the Earth. Being your mother is one of the greatest gifts of my life. It makes me push harder each day so that I can be the best example of what loving yourself enough to be healthy means.

Love Yourself. Love Your Life. Love God.

COPYRIGHT

Cover Photo by Lifestoryfoto

Author Photo by Lifestoryfoto

Graphics/Art by NelsonArtistry

ISBN-13: 978-1542469791

Published in the United States of America

INSIDE | HEALTHYLOVING

1 | *Me*

2 | *Myself*

3 | *I*

4 | *Love*

5 | *Forgiveness*

6 | *Faith*

7 | *Fitness*

8 | *Food*

PREFACE

Many moons ago, I struggled with low self-esteem. I was skinny, wore glasses, had buck teeth, and felt like I never fit in anywhere. I always marched to my own drum, but never embraced what that meant. I wanted to be different, yet didn't value those differences. I believe my "growing up" began when I went through my divorce and began a relationship with God. This is when I started to seek the purpose for my life. I guess staying connected to God allowed me to have that epiphany. It was a point where I understood that my life was important and had a purpose. I didn't need to be like anyone else. I just had to be me. All I had to do was live the purpose that God set out for me. I continue to push forward, even today, but the reality is I'm still a work in progress. In fact, learning to love yourself is a life-long process.

CHAPTER 1

M E

"Love yourself first and everything else falls into line. You really have to love yourself to get anything done in this world."

- Lucille Ball

My goal for this book is to inspire. It's not a "self-help" book, but something to help guide you along your journey toward wellness. This book is not intended to be the answer to your life-long questions. I'm not some perfect health coach who has all the answers. I continue to struggle every day, just like everyone else. Along my journey toward wellness, however, I've picked up a few things that may help you get to where you're trying to go.

Every single one of us is born with a purpose. I do not believe for one second that God intended for us to live in pain and misery. Sure, life is unfair, unjust, and sometimes downright cruel, but we must believe that the pain we experience serves a purpose.

The interesting thing about your purpose is, that's where you'll find your happiness. As a health coach, I can't figure this out for you, but I can help provide you with the tools to help you get there. Being happy starts within. It's a place where you've tended to all your issues surrounding your mind, body, and soul. A place where you have peace and feel good about the skin you're in. Each person must put the work in on him/herself. You must figure out how to motivate yourself. Sure, I can facilitate key motivational techniques to help you, but, ultimately, you must be sufficiently motivated to change your behavior/lifestyle. What is your carrot stick? What is going to get you to put the pedal to the metal?

I'm not a licensed psychologist or doctor, so you may take the contents of these pages with a grain of salt. I just know what it feels like to be broken. I've stood on a ledge with no hope or faith in my life. I've looked in the cabinets and not known how I was going to feed my boys. I remember a couple of years back when I was going through my divorce. I had a new apartment and a pile of bills to go with it. I tried to pretend that everything was fine, but the truth was that I had overextended myself financially. I was living paycheck to paycheck, and had payday loans out the ying-yang. I had a job, but did not make enough money to pay my bills. I was trying to save face from the divorce by not asking anyone for help. I was telling myself that, *"I don't need anyone. I can do this on my own."* Well, to be quite honest with you, that was dangerous and damaging self-talk. I'll never forget the moment when I came home from work and went to the cabinets to make dinner. There was NOTHING in the cabinets. I didn't even have a bag of rice. I wasn't managing my money and I couldn't even feed my children. I have never felt so helpless in my life. I couldn't believe I was putting my children through this. They deserved a whole lot better than how I was managing my life.

Early the next morning, I went out to my patio and cried out to God. I didn't know what else to do, but pray. As long as I live, I'll never forget that moment of despair. I put my pride before my children. A few hours later, my father called me. It was like God immediately intervened and saved me. **There truly is POWER in**

prayer! I knew I had to let go of my pride and allow my parents to help me. I could no longer do this by myself, not if I wanted better for the boys. Through all the worry and unknown, I became vulnerable to my truth and allowed my parents to help me. I'm thankful to have had their support through that period of my life. I know there are many out here who don't have that same opportunity.

We will go through many trials in life. You may not believe it during the storm, but you will come out of your pain tougher than you were before. What's that saying? *"Whatever doesn't kill you simply makes you stronger."* In time, you will come out of darkness. It seemed like I was never going to get out of the black hole I put myself in. I could see the light, but I didn't know how to get there.

We have this crazy illusion that our lives are supposed to be painless, problem-free, and a magical fairy tale full of love and wealth. Well, I hate to tell you the bad news, but life doesn't happen that way. Life will grow you and show you many things, but it won't be easy or perfect. There will be good, and there will be bad. We must learn to value who we are and appreciate all that has been given to us in spite of what we face. Unfortunately, a few of us never learn to love the skin we're in and can't understand how blessed we truly are. That was *me*. As a teenager, I knew I was "different." I didn't want to be like everyone else, but, at the same time, I didn't love my differences. I didn't love the skin I was in. I became overly critical of myself, which caused more harm than good. I second guessed everything I did, which created a multitude of insecurities.

My idea for this book is to share my insight, thoughts, encouragement, and perhaps help someone change his/her behavior to become his/her best self. Helping others get healthy has manifested itself beyond my wildest imagination. It brings me great joy to see people learn to love themselves enough to get healthy. Your health involves more than just going to the gym and eating better. It involves taking care of those demons and finding true peace within. Being healthy is making sure your mind, body, and spirit are being loved in a way God intended. If I can help one person begin to make positive changes in his/her life, then I'm accomplishing my purpose. I'm rooting for you to reach your next level of greatness. Think of me as your very own personal cheerleader. *GO, [Insert Your Name Here], GO!*

"Hi, My name is Coach Robbin and I'm a social media-holic." (The first step toward wellness is to know your strengths and weaknesses, HA!). HealthyLoving was born when I started sharing many of my thoughts on Facebook and Instagram. The name came to me in a dream one night. I began to share fitness challenges and nutritional tidbits to help others get healthy. Doing so changed my life. I knew this was a passion and, to my surprise, it made me happy. I pray that my posts have helped or reached people who needed that extra push. Initially, my hope was to give people better insight toward having a better life, or a simple positive message in having a better day.

So, how can I help you in this book? I'm not sure that I can help or motivate you, but, at the very least, I hope to inspire you. Throughout the following chapters, you will notice little love notes, which are intended to be helpful tips to think about during your journey toward healthyloving. I'm not saying that any of this will

change your life, but it's what helped me move toward MY best self,

so I hope it does the same for you. This is my testimony to you.

CHAPTER 2

MYSELF

"The only person who can pull me down is myself, and I'm not going to let myself pull me down anymore."

- C. JoyBell C.

We're born with unique gifts and talents that separate us from everyone else. Yet, for some strange reason, we focus on everyone else's gifts, but our own. Many of us do not believe in ourselves enough to execute our gifts. If you can sing, draw, write poetry, or have a knack in technology, it is important for you to develop your talents and gifts. It is a privilege to be born with a gift and it is your responsibility to use it.

Some of the happiest people are doing something they are passionate about. Many successful people profit from their passion. Your God-given gifts are intended to be shared with others on this Earth. Your gift allows the light within you to fulfill its purpose: to shine and bring joy to someone else's life. It's the circle of life. Our gifts help the world go around. Start thinking about what types of

passions or talents you have. What areas or types of things make

you happy? How are some ways that you can contribute to society or

the world to make it a better place?

Jot down 3 things that you like doing or sharing with

other people (This exercise will help you identify what some of

your passions may be).

1.

2.

3.

When we start focusing on helping others, it takes the focus

away from our own pain and misery. One activity that helped me

during my journey toward healthyloving was to look *myself* in the

mirror. Look at yourself in the mirror for three minutes. I want

you to take observation of a few things. What do you notice first?

What does it feel like looking at yourself? Are you happy or sad?

You might not be able to stand there for very long. There might be a level of discomfort, but please don't step away from the mirror. Continue to look deep at yourself and see what you discover.

Underneath those physical layers, recognize years of pain, neglect, and memories from the past. You may feel uneasy and want to step away from the mirror, but don't do it. Stay and face your truth. Accept it and own it. Take a hard look in the mirror to reveal your hidden truths. You know that old saying, "The truth will set you free!" There is nothing more powerful than the ability to be truthful with oneself. Many of us need to be honest with ourselves first before we can do anything else in life. Learning to love yourself begins with looking at and accepting the person in the mirror.

Know that each of us is born to do, be, love, and/or help someone or something. Our existence is bigger than ourselves and it is far bigger than the pain that we hold on to. At the beginning of my healing, I had to figure out why I was the way I was. I guess deep down, I never thought I was beautiful. I was constantly searching for someone to tell me I was. You must be open and willing to understand who you are. Learn why you make the choices you make. Being self-aware will help in the repair and recovery of your heart.

Many of us suppress our pain, go on with life, and never deal with whatever trauma or disappointment that happened to us. You may try and hide from it, but pain has this funny way of resurfacing in our lives. We hang onto pain, which keeps us connected to the past. The great thing about the past is...it's gone. You can't go back. It doesn't exist anymore. When something bad happens to you, it doesn't mean you're supposed to live in misery for the rest of your life.

God has this beautiful way of replacing what we've lost with people and things so much bigger and better than before. Be open to receiving them! You can't receive what God has planned for your future if you're still looking back at your past.

What do you want for your life? Do you want to lose weight? Do you want to exercise more? Do you need to stop drinking or smoking? Do you need to learn how to eat better? What are your specific goals that will help you get you to where you want to go in

life?

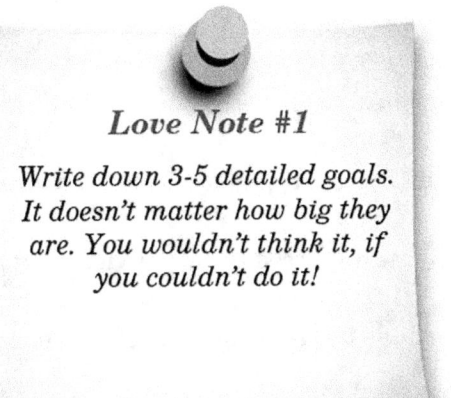

Love Note #1

*Write down 3-5 detailed goals.
It doesn't matter how big they
are. You wouldn't think it, if
you couldn't do it!*

Take a moment and write down 3-5 goals that you would

like to accomplish for your life. "Claim it, see it, and believe it!"

Write down 3-5 goals:

1.

2.

3.

4.

5.

OK, so we claimed our goals when we wrote them down. Now we just need to see them. So, how do we see them when we haven't received or accomplished them yet? We visualize them.

During my healing process, I read a book called, "The Secret," by Rhonda Byrne. It's an amazing book about the laws of attraction. Ms. Byrne discussed the art of visualization and how your vision can manifest into reality. After reading "The Secret," I immediately created a *vision board*...and it completely changed my life! I incorporated a couple of pictures into a PowerPoint slide to match goals that I had for my life. I added pictures representing all my goals and priorities, including God, college diploma, pretty smile (at that time, my teeth needed orthodontic treatment), dream home, career, and what I wanted my body to look like. I saved this as my screensaver on my laptop and saw the vision every day. I'm still working toward accomplishing a couple of those items, but it's amazing how my life has evolved. It's overwhelming when I think about the growth and change in my life. Everything that I've envisioned for my life started coming to fruition!

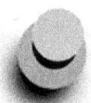

Love Note #2
Create a Vision Board. Take
your goals from Note #1 and
make them visual. Use
pictures, words or quotes to
make your vision a reality.
Place your vision board...
see it everyday!

Create your own mini vision board. Incorporate your passions, goals, and dreams. Go for what you want! Use words or quotes to represent the BIG picture. Share your vision board on social media with hashtag #HealthyLoving!

"And the LORD answered me: 'Write the vision; make it
plain on tablets, so he may run who reads it."
(Habakkuk 2:2, English Standard Version [ESV])

Finally, you must believe it. We claim to believe in the power and glory of God, but for some reason, we can't stop ourselves from worrying. Do we really believe in God, or do we say we do just to say it? You must believe it before you can receive it. Know that your change will happen. You must understand that not everything will happen right now, but it will happen in God's time. God is working and making things happen for you. So, while God is working, you should be working on your goals and positioning yourself. You can't sustain weight loss by going to the local buffet every weekend. You must take an active part in your life. When I was living paycheck to paycheck, being in the club or bar every weekend became a priority over bettering myself. I wasn't positioning myself for my situation to change. Instead of saving money or using it to further my education, I spent it on having fun.

We all have a choice in life, but we must also understand that every choice has a consequence. I'm not sure why many of us choose the hard road to travel. Perhaps it's just an experience that we all must go through. I know that my priority was to have fun and live in the moment. I think you can still do all of that, but if your priorities aren't aligned with your goals, the path to success becomes much more difficult than it needs to be. If you're not in the right position, it makes it harder for you to find God and all that He has for you.

CHAPTER 3

I

"You have been criticizing yourself for years, and it hasn't worked.
Try approving of yourself and see what happens."

- Louise L. Hay

So how do we maintain a loving, healthy relationship with ourselves? The best healing agent or medicine is a relationship with God. He said, "*I* am." He really is. Never in a million, trillion, kuh-billion years would I see me writing this book right now. When I think of all the things that have transpired over the last five years, I just throw my hands up! Wow!!! **Nothing but God!** He can make a complete change and turn your whole situation and mindset around!

Who am I? I'm a daughter, mother of two handsome young men, sister, aunt, and friend to many. Most importantly, I am a child of God. I have a purpose that God has set forth for me, and it's up to me to follow his path. My journey in life has led me to all sorts of different paths. I've had jobs to make ends meet but never a career where I was truly "happy". I've always been the type of person who wanted to help others and becoming a Health and Wellness Coach naturally fit. I thrived when I started learning about nutrition. I was excited when I was able to share wellness information to friends and family. I stayed connected to God and my "light" began to shine. As I began to heal, I wanted to help others heal. My passion became my purpose.

I know that, to this day, I am my own worst critic. I am super hard on myself, especially when I make a mistake or mess up. The negative talk we sometimes give ourselves limits our progress. Positive self-talk is filled with encouragement, compassion, and non-judgement. Start paying attention to your thoughts and how you talk to yourself. Stop telling yourself what you "can't" do and start thinking about what you "can" do. When I hear someone say, "I can't" do something, I politely reply, "You mean you won't do something." There's a difference. Words are powerful. How we speak to ourselves determines our outcome. Work on replacing words that limit you like "but" or "can't" and replace them with words that reflect opportunity, such as "and" or "can."

Whatever challenges you face, you can't get through them alone. Your belief in God will change your circumstances, outlook, and choices. I recently had the pleasure of reading, "The Daniel Plan," by Pastor Rick Warren. Let me just say, what an AMAZING book this is! It's a wonderful guide, showing us how to live a healthier and better life through a relationship with God. Pastor Warren stated that you can't face goals or challenges by yourself. You can't lose weight just by sheer willpower. You need God because only He can provide you the strength that you need to get you through it all.

I'm not saying that going to church every Sunday will fix everything. There are many people who go to church every Sunday and don't apply a single word of it to their Monday-through-Saturday lives. Many of us just aren't ready to apply His Word to our lives every day. Maybe it's a commitment or control thing, but we're just not ready to give that up. I do believe that there's a healing that takes place in church. A lot of young people today are turned off by the idea of church and religion. Why? I'm not sure if it's because of the hypocrisy displayed in the media or the idea of someone else telling you what to believe. I'm not willing to base my faith or life on what humans do. If Jesus decided to physically show up at my church one Sunday morning, I'd be super upset that I missed Him. HA! I just know it helps me be in position. *Are you in position?*

I attend church because I'm broken. To sustain good health, you must work on the "whole" person. Sure, the body and mind are important, but your spiritual mindset plays a key role in keeping you healthy. We're all broken and I identify church as a place to get whole. It's a place to share in the worship of God and fellowship with other broken believers. This life is not just about you; it's about the person hurting next to you. How can you be a light and blessing to someone else? Everyone who attends church has issues (including the minister/pastor/priest) and it's the belief and love of

God that will heal us all. Everyone who enters those church doors has a broken spirit. No one is perfect, except the God we serve. We heal best when we support one another, so why not begin your healing with the best doctor you know? He is the supreme healer!

It takes time to achieve spiritual maturity; it's not something that can be forced. When people are ready to make the commitment, they will. I'm not forcing you to have a relationship with God. It's a suggestion, in case you don't already have one. I'm not pushing some hidden religious agenda; I'm just testifying to what worked best for me. Get to know Him. Have a personal relationship with Him. Study the Bible. It contains all sorts of guidance to healthier living. Be consistent in your worship. I talk to Him every morning during my commute to work. That's my quiet time with Him and we have the best conversations!

Once you start making time for Him, your purpose will start to unfold before your eyes. I think the best thing we can do as believers is to learn as much about God as we can. We will grow daily until the day we leave this Earth. We will learn new things about God's grace and mercy, not just during periods of suffering.

God's love will help you maintain a healthyloving relationship with

yourself and others. Trust His plan for your life. Be patient. It will

be beyond your wildest imagination, but you must believe in God

and in yourself.

Love Note #3

*Establish a relationship with
God if you haven't already.
Believe in something higher
than yourself. Trust that
your end is his only
beginning. God first, your busy
schedule second!*

CHAPTER 4

L O V E

"To love oneself is the beginning of a life-long romance."
- Oscar Wilde

Depending on what version of the Bible you read, the word "love" appears 300 times in both the Old Testament and New Testament. Love is something we crave, yet it's the last thing that we completely give to ourselves. God is love and if we are willing to love each other, we are acknowledging our Holy Father.

Loving yourself is demonstrated by how you treat and value yourself. As a young teen, I didn't understand or know how to love myself. I didn't value myself. Thinking back on those times, all I wanted was affirmation that I was important. My self-esteem was low and my choices reflected that. I can remember not ever wanting to smile before I got braces. I always hid my smile because I didn't view myself as beautiful with the smile I had. After I got my braces off, you couldn't stop me from cheesing. Nothing but teeth! I've made so many mistakes trying to rush through life, trying to be something that I wasn't. Not finishing college early on was a huge mistake, but I know that it shaped me into the woman I am today. I was young and I wasn't in a healthy place where I could make good choices. I was searching for love in all the wrong places and never once learned how to love myself first.

My dad always told me, "A good man wants a God-fearing, confident, and goal-oriented woman." I truly think this is the secret to receiving your mate. Don't search for him/her. Work on yourself first. Focus on your goals and dreams. Deal with your baggage. Be the person whom you want in your life. If you're broken, who do you think you will attract? You can't go into a relationship expecting the other person to carry your baggage. Relationships work when you have two "whole" individuals coming together complementing one another. Like a magnet. Once you become it, you attract it. #ImAWitness.

We all make mistakes. Unfortunately, those mistakes tend to shape the course of our lives. I tell my boys all the time, "The choices you make today will impact your tomorrow." I'm not saying that loving yourself will prevent you from making mistakes, as mistakes are inevitable and necessary for growth. I'm saying that your choices are a result of how you feel inside. Your actions reflect your feelings. God is involved in everything we face, including the good, bad, and the ugly. He only wants the best for us. He does, however, allow us to experience tragedy so that we will learn to depend on Him, and lean on His grace and strength.

So, how do you begin to heal and learn to love yourself? You first must forgive yourself—for your mistakes, choices, and behavior. I told you earlier that the past is gone. We can't fix it. It happened. The great thing about today is that you are alive. Stop living present in your pain. It is a blessing to wake up every morning with another opportunity to make life better! Amen? How divine and awesome is that? Who gives second chances like that?

I used to play this wonderful role back in the day. Oh, my goodness! I think I would've won best actress of the year for this role. You know that role we often play? The "victim!" Many people these days can play that part to perfection. *Merriam Webster's Dictionary* defines "victim" as "someone who is deceived or cheated, as by his or her own emotions or ignorance, by the dishonesty of others."

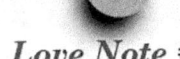

Love Note #4

Learn to forgive yourself. For whatever issues, mistakes, neglect or ignorance that you are holding close to your heart. Forgive yourself. Let go of the past and move forward. Pray on it and be FREE of the pain!

Playing victim prevents us from seeing the light at the end of the tunnel. It gives in to our fears. If you fall victim to this mindset, you will never feel better about yourself. Complaining and crying only creates confusion. There is no solution when there is confusion.

Sometimes being the victim allows us to not move forward because we want to punish the person who hurt us, that "eye for an eye" mentality. The truth is, your happiness should never be dependent on what someone else does or doesn't do to or for you.

Everyone will experience pain or heartache at some point in their life. Take comfort in knowing that it's only temporary. Have you ever experienced a bee sting or been given a shot? It stings for a minute, and then after a while, you don't feel the pain or even remember that you were stung. Be honest with yourself for a moment. When you looked in the mirror, did you like what you saw? I know that every time I look in the mirror, I focus on the negative things I see, including all my flaws, from my nose to my rolls! We automatically see negative things and start comparing ourselves to an image or version of what we think we should look like. We must learn to love ourselves as we are. Know that you are beautifully made, most precious and beautiful to God. He wants you to be able to love yourself as much as He loves you.

There's a difference in being content with who we are and being down right negligent. There are things that we do have control over and can fix ourselves. Being overweight and unhealthy can be prevented. Focus on the things that you do have power to work on, such as your weight, appearance, job, or education. You have control over those items and can change your circumstances. However, it will require dedication, commitment, and effort on your part. It won't be easy. Nothing in life ever worth it is. When you can be honest with yourself, that's when the change and healing takes place. It won't happen right away, but it will happen. Believe that you can be happy and start loving the person God intended you to be.

Start a "Kudos Section" in your journal. Every day, capture what great things others say about you. Go back and read those comments once a month, to remind yourself how GREAT and wonderful you really are!

Write down 3 GREAT compliments that you've received in the

last month (work, home, social media, etc.):

1.

2.

3.

My question to you is, "Do you LOVE yourself?" Embrace

who you are, the skin that you're in, and position yourself to receive

all that God has for you. Think of life as an extravagant present

that is ready to be unwrapped. Get to work and start unwrapping

it.

CHAPTER 5

FORGIVENESS

*"The weak can never forgive. Forgiveness is the
attribute of the strong."*

- Gandhi

The Bible instructs us to love thy neighbor. Many people

have a hard time understanding what that means. You can't just

love some people or people who are only like you. It means the

entire human race. Let's hypothetically say that someone did you

wrong. Do you know how much energy is involved in "hating" or

"hurting" someone who hurt you? Such energy is a never-ending

cycle, taking up so much space in your life.

We have only a limited amount of time here on Earth. Being

upset wastes so much time and energy on something so

meaningless. Negative energy creates stress and drama, which are major contributors to chronic illnesses. Why give someone or something so much power in your life? Why not be free from all the pain in your heart? I think we get caught up and feed off the hate. We don't feel good unless we know someone else feels worse. I'm not saying it's easy to let it go, because it's not. I'm just saying that letting go will bring you to a place of freedom and peace of mind. No one is going to "get over" on you. It doesn't make you a weak person by turning the other cheek. It just means that you are a forgiving person who can let things go in order to move forward. By not letting go, we hold on to the past.

There are countless stories involving cases where co-parenting went wrong. One parent is not compromising or making things difficult for the other parent. It has nothing to do with the child, but everything to do with the wrong-doing in their relationship. You can't make someone love you. If it's over, let it go and move on with your life. After my divorce, from day one, my focus was my boys and not dwelling on the pain of a failed marriage. I didn't want to live my life in constant pain and reflection on what went wrong. It didn't work out, but we have two beautiful kids from it. The end. I'm thankful that both of us can put our children first. My priorities were my boys and showing them how to resolve issues in relationships like rational human beings. Forgiveness was essential and necessary for me to move forward. I didn't want our children having mommy/daddy issues because of what their parents exposed them to.

Half of the issues many of us face today as adults, stems from what happened to us in our childhood. I was determined that I was going to maintain a healthy environment for my boys. Stop using your children as pawns and go sit down somewhere and deal with your baggage quietly. Forgiveness also means forgetting. You can't forgive unless you're willing to forget. Stop holding people hostage to your pain. Nine times out of ten, those same people who hurt you aren't even thinking about you. **Let it go!** If you're unable to bare the weight of whatever issue you hold, find someone trustworthy to whom you can release that burden from your soul.

I love observing people in restaurants who have received bad service or their food took a long time to arrive. It is amazing how little patience and what a huge amount of importance we think we have. When the food finally does arrive, the customer feels he/she's entitled to be rude to the server or manager. Crap happens. I would love to come to your job one day and go off on you for all the mistakes you make. Just once, I wish that people could walk in other people's shoes for one day. Maybe it would teach us how to have a little more empathy for one another.

Things that happen in life won't always be perfect, but how we react to them says a lot about our character. After waiting tables for many years, you learn a lot about people. There are good people in this world, and there are also people out there who truly enjoy hurting others. I decided a while ago that no one would determine or steal my joy, no matter what they tried to do to me. God's peace gives me joy in my soul. It saddens me when others are unable to let go of pain. Choosing not to forgive allows the enemy to keep you in your pain.

One benefit of forgiveness is that it gives you the ability to move forward. What good is it to hold stuff over someone's head? It's like when a child stands in a mud puddle. They look down and know it's dirty, yet they stand there and splash around, getting themselves covered in dirt. You're not going to rid yourself of the pain if you're constantly standing in it.

Think of an issue or person that you are having trouble forgiving. Write them a short paragraph describing how you would show them compassion. Describe ways that you would be kinder to them and how you will forgive them.

Forgiveness Letter: (Write a short paragraph to the person you choose to forgive)

_____

_____

_____

_____

_____

After my divorce, I focused more on the fact that I had failed at my marriage. I wasn't thinking about the fact that it was over, but, rather, that I didn't keep it together. I cared more about what others thought rather than what was best for me. How could I fail at staying married? How embarrassing having all those people at my wedding and now I'm going through a divorce! I had to get over myself if I was going to get through this. My father gave me some great advice while I was going through my divorce. He said, "Get a relationship with God. He will help you through it." For the first time in my life, I listened to him. (He'll love to see this part of the book! HA!)

I started asking God for strength, peace, guidance…and wouldn't you know it? My life began to turn around. I look back on those times and laugh at myself and mindset. I was in bad shape! I had no goals, nothing to look forward to for myself, except my kids. What on Earth had I been doing all this time? I had to take a step back and look at some of the decisions I was making. I had to be real with myself. I had to be honest. Truthfully, I needed to grow up. It was time to hold myself accountable for the bad choices I had made in my life. These choices reflected someone who was starving for love and didn't love herself. We are all emotional creatures. We rely on our emotions, instead of leaning on God. I made hasty decisions based on how I was feeling at that moment. I've grown as a person tremendously over the last few years. I like myself and I'm still working on loving myself. I reflect on the past, but I don't live there. What happened in the past may be terrible, but we live through it. There's proof of that because you are reading this wonderful book that I wrote for you! HA!

Life is a mystery. No one has all the answers, but while we're here, wouldn't you rather be happy? Don't you want to laugh? **Learn to take God seriously, but don't take yourself so seriously!** You have the choice to choose your emotions. Appreciate what/who you have and don't for one second take any of it for granted. Choose not to live in pain and sadness for the rest of your years. Forgive, forget, and go forward! Life will not be perfect. Somebody lied to you if they told you it would. Every morning we open our eyes is another day closer to the promise God has planned

for you. Use your pain as a tool and take this opportunity to give it

everything you got. It won't be easy, but you'll know that you gave

every effort at being your best self.

Love Note #5
Learn to let the small stuff go!
Next time your upset, take a
moment and observe your
emotions. Your pain does not
define who you are, your
triumph through the mess
does! Forgive yourself. Forgive
others. Move on. Live!

Forgive others so that you can lead a happy and stress-free

life. The moment you're able to forgive, the better you will feel

inside.

CHAPTER 6

FAITH

*"Faith is taking the first step even when you don't
see the whole staircase."*
- Dr. Martin Luther King, Jr.

It's simple. Without **faith**, you won't make it in this life. You

could probably exist, but you wouldn't be living. Whatever your

heart desires, you have the power and strength within you to make

the changes that you need to achieve those desires. Many people

battle with weight, nutrition, and exercise. You can't do any of it

without God. People think willpower is all they need to help them

through their change in lifestyle. God provides us with the strength

we need, yet we generally try and do this big change without Him.

Have you ever wondered why you never stuck to any of your trendy

diets?

As I mentioned earlier, creating a vision board worked beyond my wildest imagination. It changed how I saw myself and all the negative things that I was speaking into my life. You can't have a positive life with a negative mindset. By creating a vision board, I was speaking goals into my life. Put your vision board somewhere you can see it daily. You will instill within yourself the faith that it will happen.

A few items on my vision board have already come into reality. I can't explain it. I don't even know how it happened, but it did. It may have been my faith in God. It could've been how I started positioning myself. Those are the only explanations that I can come up with. I can't even explain half of it really, as it's truly a magnificent mystery. A relationship with God changed the course of my life. It strengthened who I was inside and I began to have faith that it would all work out.

When you have faith, you are giving God the "OK" to make your life better. It's like opening a window and receiving all the goodness that God has planned for your life. You must make that choice to let Him in, and not only when you're in trouble. For instance, let's say you're a person who rarely prays and goes to church on special occasions like Easter or Christmas. One day you're on a plane. The plane begins to experience serious turbulence. I can almost guarantee you there will be some level of prayer, or an "Oh God! Get me through this" moment. It's like we only call on Him or have a relationship with Him when we need Him. We stop dealing with family and friends when they do that, so imagine how God feels. This must be a daily relationship, like the one you have with your kids, pets, and parents. He protected and shielded you from harm's way on the plane because He loves you. Just imagine a life where you have a consistent and connected relationship with Him. #BeyondYourImagination.

Find quiet time with Him, whether it's early in the morning before everyone gets up, or before bed, but talk to Him. Let Him into your heart and tell Him where you are trying to go. Trust that He will help you get there. You don't have to be this super religious person to talk to God. All you need to do is just speak from your heart and make time for Him. How do you stay connected?

My quiet place is my walk-in closet. I pray, I plan, and I prepare. Going to this quiet place allows me to stay connected and leaves me with so much peace. Another helpful way that I stay connected is walking with God. Take time to stroll your neighborhood or a safe trail. Get outside and talk to God! Your neighbors may start looking at you like you're crazy, but get your walk on! Speak from your heart. This form of meditation is amazing! You will start to become more aware of the different sounds, smells, and air around you. This is an opportunity to appreciate what's around you. It's truly an awakening experience!

CHAPTER 7

FITNESS

"Our growing softness, our increasing lack of physical fitness,
is a menace to our security."
- John F. Kennedy

You must move your body! You were given two arms, two legs, and a head that turns. They are supposed to move, not sit on the couch watching TV all day. One thing that I'd like you to understand is that your body is a gift from God. Why do we choose to mismanage it so much? We take care of our children and our pets better than we take care of ourselves. It amazes me to hear people say that they hate to walk or run when there are millions of people in wheelchairs who wish they had just one opportunity to move their legs again. We take SO MUCH for granted!

Physical *fitness* is necessary for your well-being. It reduces risks and prevents many diseases. Exercise can improve your state of being. Think about how much energy you have and better you feel after a nice walk or workout. Some of you may be out of breath and need a minute to recover, but for the most part, you have more energy from working out. For some reason, when we have something detrimental or bad happen to us, we stop moving. It's like if we sit in misery, then we can continue to punish ourselves with whatever went wrong. Stop it! Stop it! Stop it! As my mama told me, "The best revenge against anything bad happening to you is your success."

I've been thin for most of my life. (Don't think because I've been thin that I haven't had my own issues with self-image.) Life after kids somehow changed the thin version of Robbin. It brought unhealthy eating, added curves, and low amounts of energy. In the past forty-three years, I've never had to struggle with my weight until now. Life after 40 left me with a slower metabolism and unwanted fat in my mid-section. I love cake, donuts, fried chicken, fried fish, macaroni and cheese, and mashed potatoes and gravy. SIGH! Although I'm a health coach, I have my weaknesses, just like everyone else. In fact, "The way my fat in my mid-section is set up

(Kevin Hart joke)" ... I know my fat isn't going to go away unless I change my behavior. I have to want the change and be disciplined enough to say "No" when I want to eat unhealthy. However, we still need to be kind to ourselves when we do fall off the bike. Beating ourselves up because we ate the entire bag of Spicy Doritos (this is all hypothetical; HA!) will not encourage or promote a healthier lifestyle for your mind, body, and spirit.

We will have good days and bad days. On those bad days, we still need to stay active. Get outside and enjoy the fresh air. Walk in the mall, go up and down the steps, take your dog out for a walk, but MOVE. Stay active. Don't let your bad days defeat your progress.

You are here to manage the gift that God gave to you, so be responsible with it. Once I got that in my head, the choices I made about fitness and nutrition began to change. I still eat terrible at times, but I'm better than I used to be. Quite frankly, I just started to care. You have the same ability within you. You don't have to care or follow any of my advice, but if you don't care, you won't see change. Join a gym, work out at home, or walk in your neighborhood. Discuss fitness goals, challenges, and limitations with your doctor. Strive for exercise to be a part of your daily routine. Once I joined the gym and found a regimen that worked for me and my abilities, I began to see results. I started to fall in love with my body and now you can't keep me out of the mirror. I also noticed an increase in energy after working out. I could complete chores and deal with my crazy boys after a long day.

A great website and resource for finding programs and exercise routines is Bodybuilding.com. It's a great site to help the beginner achieve personal daily goals. It also has a mobile app to keep track of programs you complete daily. You can search for

workout programs that are specific to duration, age, and gender.

Try this fitness routine. You can do this every morning. It will ensure you are getting movement/fitness in every day.

WAKE UP: STRETCH for 3 minutes. Ground your thoughts and breathe through each movement.

AM: 10 Jumping Jacks or Side Steps

5 Push Ups on Knees or wall (if you have bad knees)

10 Squats

10 Crunches

NOON: Walk at a fast pace for 10 minutes. (Outside or inside a building)

PM: 10 Jumping Jacks or Side Steps

10 High Knees

5 Push Ups on Knees or wall (if you have bad knees)

10 Calf Raises

EVENING: Walk at a fast pace for 10 minutes
(Outside or inside a building)

Look at that! You completed twenty minutes of cardio without even stepping foot inside a gym. A few simple exercises like these will get your heart rate elevated and boost energy levels.

You must work for what you want in life. Everything is not given to you. I can't do this for you. All I can do is share what worked for me and, perhaps, provide motivation or insight into your own journey toward wellness. There is no "one-size-fits-all" plan for health. All I can do is suggest tools and resources that will help you get there yourself. Learn to empower yourself. Do your own research. When in doubt, Google it. *Learn so you can live.* After you've begun to heal, be sure to start sharing your story with others. **Each One. Teach One.**

CHAPTER 8

FOOD

"There is no such thing as junk food. There is junk. There is food."

- Dr. Mark Hyman

Food—the final chapter! It's one of the biggest reasons we are so unhealthy. We are emotional eaters. We eat because that's what we're taught to do. We're not taught to eat for nourishment or to fuel our bodies. We're taught to eat for satisfaction and flavor. We eat because we associate food with self-gratification. You may think you're hungry, but you're not. That's just your mind (sugar) playing tricks on you. You must fuel your body with the proper nutrition to achieve optimal performance.

This country is in a state of information overload when it comes to nutrition and fitness. Do your own research and don't just take a fitness coach or a doctor's word for it. Everyone has the "formula for success" to getting healthy. No matter what advice or information you research, do what is best for YOUR body. A good general rule that I like to keep is this: Balance is key. If you're extremely disciplined, then you won't have a problem staying on target. However, if you're an emotional eater, like me, you will need to learn how to establish some balance and discipline methods.

How do I try to maintain balance? I drink mostly water (carbon-filtered); try to eat more vegetables than starches; limit my meat, fruit, and sugar intake; and I make sure to eat breakfast every morning. If that sounds difficult, then I don't know what else to tell you.

DO NOT DENY YOURSELF! One thing that I've noticed over the years is that when we're on a diet, many of us will deny ourselves foods that we may crave or want. As I stated earlier, we are emotional eaters. Unless you have learned to eat for fuel, don't put yourself through the stress. When we become over critical of ourselves after eating the entire box of donuts, we stop trying. The goal is to keep going, not quit. Follow your nutrition plan, but don't beat yourself up after you fall short. You may have to start all over again, but changing behaviors takes time and it's not going to happen overnight Keep your eye on the goal and keep swimming.

I'd like to spend this next section discussing five basic tips that can help you get started toward better nutrition. You can take it or leave it, but I think these areas are a great start to helping you toward any weight-loss goals that you may have.

1.   *Sodas.*

They are bad for you! Stop drinking them! Many studies have shown where sodas are related to severe health risks, linking them to disease, obesity, and sickness. Did you know that the average American drinks approximately 56 gallons of soda a year? The more soda that you drink, it changes the dynamic of your taste buds. It takes away from the enjoyment of eating healthier foods. Drinking sodas makes you crave sweeter foods. It tells you that you're hungry when you're not, which makes you EAT more. "Well, I just drink diet sodas." Diet sodas contain artificial sweeteners that still put you at risk. Diet drinks are linked to disease, belly fat, high blood sugar, and cholesterol. So, don't think that drinking "diet" gives you this free pass toward healthier living.

If you are trying to lose weight, drinking sodas is not the ticket. They are high in calories and have no nutritional value whatsoever. The carbonation in sodas binds fat cells, thus slowing down the fat-burning process and your digestion. Think about this question: "What is natural about the substance I'm drinking?" I can go on and on about the harm that sodas will do to your body, but I will just end with this: They're bad for you. If it's not water or an herbal tea, then you shouldn't drink it.

2. *Sugar.*

I wasn't aware of how bad sugar was until I read, "The Daniel Plan." All I can say is that this book opened my eyes to so many facts about nutrition. Do your research and know what you're consuming. Remember this: "Where there is sugar, you will find disease." Empower yourself to learn about foods that enter your body. Did you know that sugar is nine times more addictive than heroin? Now it makes sense why I can eat a whole box of Krispy

Kremes! You can't have just one, especially if the "red light" is on! We must learn how to read our ingredient labels. Sugar has so many different names that it can be misleading when a label says, "no sugar added," yet in the list of ingredients, it's under a completely different name. This explains why we are at such high risk for disease and obesity. Unfortunately, many of us would rather eat fast, processed foods than cook real foods at home. "Eating healthy is so expensive." At the end of the year, how much will you spend in medical bills, co-pays, or prescription meds? Avoid those medical costs and make the investment in your nutrition. I've seen instances where cutting sugar has significantly lowered blood pressure dosages, or gotten people completely off their blood pressure medicine. Food is medicine. What we eat is what we become.

Farmer's markets are an inexpensive way to get fresh produce and seasonable vegetables. Learn what your community has to offer. Begin to tap into those resources instead of grabbing the easiest. It could save your life in the long run.

If you have a big family, it can be discouraging planning healthier meals. The costs up front appear to be extremely high in comparison to buying processed foods. There are ways that you can save money and prepare real foods for your family. Buy what you need for the week. More times than not, vegetables and fruit go bad because our taste buds change. Buy frozen veggies and fruits to keep them from going bad so quickly. Try fixing casseroles or crock pot meals to save time and money. Bake granola bars or prep veggies for snacks, which can go a long way. Chips and cookies may seem cheaper than fruit, but aren't they gone in the same amount of time? (At least in my household they are.)

Learn to prep and plan your meals. Start out by developing some consistency to your healthy eating. Keep it simple so you can sustain it. We get all this energy and excitement at the prospect of eating healthy and create a lot of complex recipes. Those recipes call for many ingredients (which can be expensive). You're less likely to stay consistent with eating healthy if it's complicated or expensive. We like fast, easy, and cheap. So, keep your meals that way, just healthier.

3. *Vegetables.*

Another favorite way you can eat healthy on a budget is growing your own food. There is something very spiritual about growing your own food. Planting seeds, growing, and the harvest! Sounds like the circle of life to me. Vegetables are God's gifts to us, yet they're the one thing that most of us fail to eat. Veggies are low in fat and contain zero cholesterol. They are the best medicine known to man. Vegetables provide the necessary nutrients for our bodies to be at their best performance. These wonderful little creatures help prevent us from getting diseases, strokes, and cancer. They contain fiber needed to improve your bowels and keep your skin, hair, and teeth healthy.

It's recommended that we eat 7-9 servings of vegetables daily. I think I used to prepare like 1-2 servings per week, removing all the nutrients from overcooking. I'm a product of good ole' southern cooking. My mother will put her FOOT in some

Mustard Greens! Woo! Growing up, vegetables in my house were heavily seasoned and with some type of pork in it. Although that bacon grease may "turn up" that cabbage, it adds no nutritional value whatsoever. Sure, it may taste good, but there are other ways you can flavor your veggies. There are a lot of simple and easy recipes to prepare vegetables. You don't have to boil all the green out of the broccoli for it to taste good. Use fresh seasonings and herbs, healthy oils, and roast or grill your veggies.

Check out this favorite southern dish made healthy:

Sautéed Cabbage

- *4 cups of shredded cabbage*
- *2 tbsp. olive oil or grapeseed oil*
- *3-4 cloves garlic, minced*
- *Pinch of crushed red pepper*
- *Salt and Pepper to taste*

Place cabbage in large bowl and soak in water. Heat sauté pan and add oil. Add garlic. Add soaked cabbage to pan and toss for 10-12min. Throw pinch of crushed red pepper. Add Salt and Pepper to taste. Put lid on and continue to toss until tender.

4. *Fruits.*

Fruits are another God-given gift. They provide us with various nutritional benefits and vitamins needed for optimal health. Fruit is seasonal and we should eat moderate amounts. People get over zealous with their weight-loss journey and the first thing they do is grab a huge bowl of fruit. You need more than fruit and a salad to begin this journey. I appreciate your progress, but, first, understand what you're eating. Creamy dressings on a salad do nothing for you, except give you added calories and sugar. That's why salads never fill you up because you haven't learned the right things to put on them. You will need a balance to your meals, including carbs, fiber, and protein. Yes, fruit contains natural sugars, but it's still made of glucose, which equals sugar. We've already determined that sugar is the devil. Sugar is BAD! Be careful with fruit smoothies and juices that are also loaded with unwanted sugars.

You must do your own research and take responsibility for your own health. The best bet is to find yourself a nutritionist who can guide you along your journey to wellness. He/she can inform you of certain foods that may affect your body that you may not even be aware of. The results of some studies have shown that our blood type is a key factor to why we react to certain foods or have excessive weight gain.

It's interesting to watch the bandwagon when there's a new diet or detox out. A quick fix for losing 20 lbs. overnight will never sustain your weight loss. A pill, shake, wrap, or supplement will do you no good until you learn to change the behavior. You will complete the challenge, go back to the unhealthy lifestyle, and end up weighing even more than before. Until you have self-awareness and get smart on nutrition, it will be a never-ending cycle of keeping the weight off.

During the week, the drive through feeds my boys. It's sad, but true. I feel so guilty when I don't cook. I buy the foods, but then I get lazy or tired and go for what's easiest. We have got to be more responsible and aware of the foods we consume. Our children eat what we provide. They are watching, learning, and repeating. We are products of our environment. To this day, I eat a lot of the same foods that I ate as a child. I can still taste that fried bologna with mustard on white bread! We must provide our children with the essential nutrients to give them optimal health. There is an alarming rate of childhood obesity and other behavioral problems stemming from too much sugar and processed foods, and not enough vegetables. I get it. Eating out can be cheaper and easier. I'm right there with you. We just have to be and do better. If not for ourselves, then for our kids.

5. *Water.*

My final tip that I'm going to leave you with is to increase your water intake. Your body needs it, plain and simple. You need water for detoxifying, metabolism, staying hydrated, and regulating your body temperature. When we drink sugary drinks, we load unwanted sugars and dehydrate our bodies. You may often experience sugar cravings. More than likely, it's because your body is dehydrated. Listen to your body. If you're thirsty, odds are you need water.

Depending on how active you are, a good rule of thumb is to drink half of your body weight in ounces. So, if you weigh 150 lbs., you should be drinking at least 75 oz. of water every day. If you can't drink that much water, at least try and get the recommended amount of 64 oz. daily. Pay attention to your urine. If it's a dark yellowish color, you should lay off other beverages and drink more water. Your urine should be a light, pale yellow. Don't get alarmed when you have to go to the bathroom every five minutes. Your body is working the way it's supposed to. Water is an agent that God provided to flush away nasty toxins from our bodies. I often hear people say, "Water has no taste." It's not supposed to have taste; it's supposed to hydrate your body. However, you can infuse water with slices of lemon, lime, or oranges to help enhance the flavor. The best part about water is that it's free, and it's a key factor toward reaching your weight-loss goals.

Let's try another activity. Before you is a *HealthyLoving* eating schedule. I want you to fill it in with what you ate for the day.

Time	Meal	Items Eaten:
6:00-7:00AM	Breakfast	Fiber –
Total ounces of Water? _____		Protein – Carbs – Good Fats -
9:30-10:00AM	AM Snack	
12:00 NOON	Lunch	Fiber –
Total ounces of Water? _____		Protein – Carbs – Good Fats -
2:30-3:00	PM Snack	
6:00-7:00	Dinner	Fiber –
Total ounces of Water? _____		Protein – Carbs – Good Fats -
8:00PM	Dessert	

Did you have any gaps? Were you on target and ate something at each period of the day? Do you feel that you got in your essential nutrients for the day? A secret to good nutrition is learning how to provide fuel and substance to your body for the entire day. Skipping breakfast or starving yourself does more harm than good. It can deprive your body of essential nutrients, slows down your metabolism, and cause your blood sugar to drop, which will kill all of your energy. Your body needs REAL food to get you through the day, and get the best performance out of you it can.

Love Note #8
Increase your vegetables, limit your fruit intake. Learn to plan and prep what foods you need to be eating on a daily basis. Get adequate amounts of water and eliminate sugary drinks to perform as your best self.

CONCLUSION

HEAL

"You can try to change in ways that allow you to be more healthy and happy, but this is done because you care about yourself, not because you are worthless or unacceptable as you are."
- Kristin Neff

You have a specific divine plan that's assigned to you. Fight for your chance to be great. Do your best to discover and figure out what that is before you leave this Earth. Time is of the essence. No one knows when their time is up. The favor is there, the resources are available, but you must want it for yourself.

Through faith, fitness and nutrition, I began to get better. I became healthy. I can't wait for you to begin to heal and start loving yourself enough to be healthy. The blessings and change will be beyond your imagination. I wish you the very best on your journey to loving yourself enough to be healthy! Be blessed!

Love and Blessings,

Coach Robbin

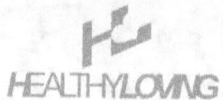
HEALTHYLOVING

ACTION GUIDE

Wellness Activity #1

Look yourself in the mirror for 3 minutes. Describe what it felt like to look at yourself in the mirror. Were you able to look at yourself for the entire 3 minutes? What types of things did you discover about yourself?

_____

_____

_____

_____

_____

_____

_____

_____

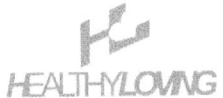
HEALTHYLOVING

ACTION GUIDE

Wellness Activity #2

Complete the below meditation exercises and journal how each of them made you feel. Share your thoughts in the 'Notes' section, in the back of the book. Will you continue to try these exercises? Did these calm or give you any peace?

Walking meditation

Take a walk with nature and focus on what's around you. No phones, no music. Just listen to the sounds around you. This is a great opportunity to talk with God!

War Room

Create a quiet space in your home where you can pray. Add pictures, quotes, Bible and other items that bring motivation and peace to your spirit. Pray for however long you need. 10-15 min. is a great start. (You'll be surprised how long you'll be in there the first time!) If you don't know how to pray, just say whatever is on your heart. Oh…and bring the tissues!

Give Thanks!

What are you thankful for? Write down 10 things that you are grateful for. On another sheet of paper, write down 5 things that you take for granted. Did those things you take for granted surprise you? Try to repeat this every day by writing at least 3 things you're grateful for and 3 things you will no longer take for granted.

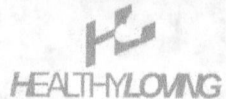

ACTION GUIDE

Wellness Activity #3

Take 1 item out of your pantry with a nutrition label that you LOVE to eat. Now read the label. List 5 of the ingredients and Google what each word means. Rule of thumb: If it has more than 5 items listed, it's not real food with any nutritional value.

Item: _____

Ingredient	*Origin/Meaning*
_____	_____
_____	_____
_____	_____
_____	_____
_____	_____

Are you comfortable consuming these ingredients now that you know the origin of their meaning? Take 5 other items from your pantry and begin to study your ingredient labels. Do you think you will begin to look at the labels before buying items in the store again?

REFERENCES

P 12; 31   Byrne, Rhonda. *The Secret*. New York: Atria, 2006.
                Print.

P 20   Merriam-Webster's Collegiate Dictionary, 2005

P 17; 31;   Warren, Richard. The Daniel plan: 40 days to a
42   healthier life. Grand Rapids, MI: Zondervan, 2013.
                Print.

P 39   http://bodyspace.bodybuilding.com/RC26."Bodybuilding
                Workouts, Exercise, and Diet."About.com Sports. N. p.,
                05 Mar. 2016. Web. 13 Jan. 2017.

P 51   The War Room. Dir. Alex Kendrick. FaithStep, Affirm
                Films, Red Sky Studios, TriStar Pictures, 2015. DVD.

NOTES

NOTES

NOTES